Repellents:

35 DIY Natural Recipes to Protect Your Family And Yourself From Mosquitos

Table of Contents

Introduction

Summer is just around the corner, and with it comes warmer days, rays of sunshine, and all kinds of outdoor fun. You know you are already working on your swimsuit body, your plans for the summer, and thinking about all the wonderful things you want to do this year.

But there's one part of summer you aren't looking forward to – and that's all the bugs.

Sure, these creatures have their purpose on this planet just like we do, but surely that purpose doesn't have to do anything with us. When it comes to the world of bugs, you know you want nothing more than to just see them leave.

You hate being bitten, stung, crawled on, and not being able to enjoy the activity you are doing for fear you are going to get invaded with pests.

Thankfully, you have come to the right place. This book is full of what you need to know to get rid of these pests in your life, and it is everything you need to ensure that they aren't going to come back. With each of these bug repellents, you have just what you need to ensure you are safe to enjoy any activity without bugs.

And to make it even better, you don't have to worry about your pets or children, either. Use only organic materials, and you are going to get everything you need to keep yourself and your family comfortable, without having to worry that you are putting anything harmful on your skin.

Make one or make them all – just discover which is your favorite and which you want to use time and time again.

Summer is meant to be enjoyed, and with these bug repellents, you are able to do that very thing.

Chapter 1 – Shoo Fly, Don't Bother Me

Picnic Partner

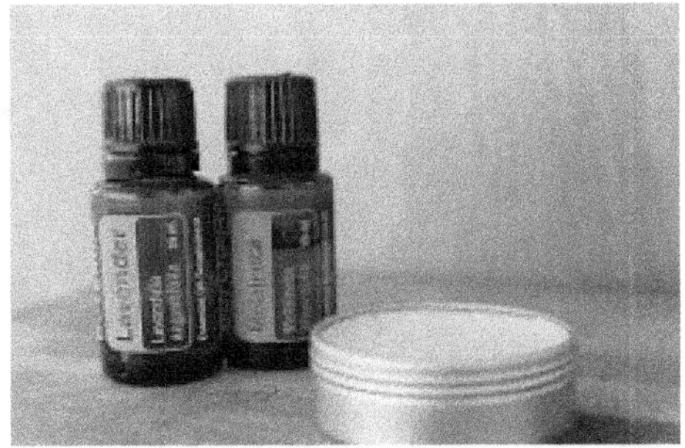

What you will need:

10 drops garlic oil

10 drops peppermint oil

½ cup water

1 tablespoon witch hazel

2 teaspoons castor oil

1 teaspoon black pepper oil

Directions:

Mix all ingredients well, then transfer into a spray bottle or spritzer. When you are ready to use, shake the bottle thoroughly each time, and generously spray the area that is currently infected, or the area you want to protect from infestation.

If you wish to use it as a repellent on yourself, simple spray your wrists and rub it around the back of your neck and behind your ears. This is not waterproof, so if you go swimming you will need to reapply.

Also reapply as needed.

No Ants in My Pants
What you will need:

10 drops peppermint oil

8 drops lemon oil

½ cup water

1 tablespoon witch hazel

2 teaspoons castor oil

1 teaspoon black pepper oil

Directions:

Mix all ingredients well, then transfer into a spray bottle or spritzer. When you are ready to use, shake the bottle thoroughly each time, and generously spray the area that is currently infected, or the area you want to protect from infestation.

If you wish to use it as a repellent on yourself, simple spray your wrists and rub it around the back of your neck and behind your ears. This is not waterproof, so if you go swimming you will need to reapply.

Also reapply as needed.

Off Limit Zone

What you will need:

10 drops clary sage oil

9 drops vetiver oil

½ cup water

1 tablespoon witch hazel

2 teaspoons castor oil

1 teaspoon black pepper oil

Directions:

Mix all ingredients well, then transfer into a spray bottle or spritzer. When you are ready to use, shake the bottle thoroughly each time, and generously spray the area that is currently infected, or the area you want to protect from infestation.

If you wish to use it as a repellent on yourself, simple spray your wrists and rub it around the back of your neck and behind your ears. This is not waterproof, so if you go swimming you will need to reapply.

Also reapply as needed.

Summer's Night

What you will need:

10 drops cinnamon oil

9 drops clove oil

½ cup water

1 tablespoon witch hazel

2 teaspoons castor oil

1 teaspoon black pepper oil

Directions:

Mix all ingredients well, then transfer into a spray bottle or spritzer. When you are ready to use, shake the bottle thoroughly each time, and generously spray the area that is currently infected, or the area you want to protect from infestation.

If you wish to use it as a repellent on yourself, simple spray your wrists and rub it around the back of your neck and behind your ears. This is not waterproof, so if you go swimming you will need to reapply.

Also reapply as needed.

Gone Fishing
What you will need:

10 drops tea tree oil

5 drops sage oil

½ cup water

1 tablespoon witch hazel

2 teaspoons castor oil

1 teaspoon black pepper oil

Directions:

Mix all ingredients well, then transfer into a spray bottle or spritzer. When you are ready to use, shake the bottle thoroughly each time, and generously spray the area that is currently infected, or the area you want to protect from infestation.

If you wish to use it as a repellent on yourself, simple spray your wrists and rub it around the back of your neck and behind your ears. This is not waterproof, so if you go swimming you will need to reapply.

Also reapply as needed.

Better Bee-leave It
What you will need:

12 drops eucalyptus oil

8 drops orange oil

½ cup water

1 tablespoon witch hazel

2 teaspoons castor oil

1 teaspoon black pepper oil

Directions:

Mix all ingredients well, then transfer into a spray bottle or spritzer. When you are ready to use, shake the bottle thoroughly each time, and generously spray the area that is currently infected, or the area you want to protect from infestation.

If you wish to use it as a repellent on yourself, simple spray your wrists and rub it around the back of your neck and behind your ears. This is not waterproof, so if you go swimming you will need to reapply.

Also reapply as needed.

Barbecues and Parties

What you will need:

10 drops lavender oil

7 drops lemon oil

½ cup water

1 tablespoon witch hazel

2 teaspoons castor oil

1 teaspoon black pepper oil

Directions:

Mix all ingredients well, then transfer into a spray bottle or spritzer. When you are ready to use, shake the bottle thoroughly each time, and generously spray the area that is currently infected, or the area you want to protect from infestation.

If you wish to use it as a repellent on yourself, simple spray your wrists and rub it around the back of your neck and behind your ears. This is not waterproof, so if you go swimming you will need to reapply.

Also reapply as needed.

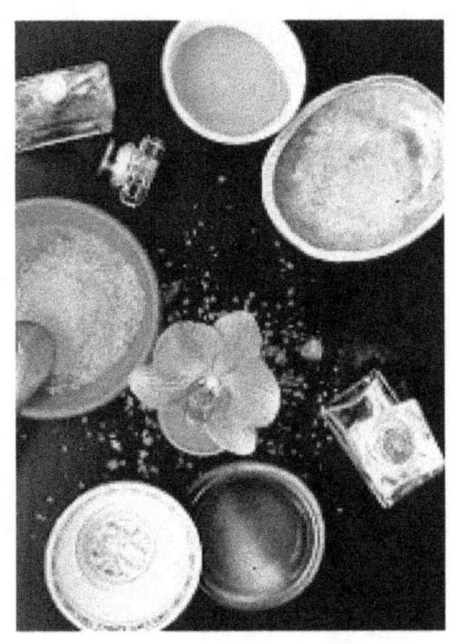

Safety Net

What you will need:

12 drops clove oil

2 drops frankincense oil

½ cup water

1 tablespoon witch hazel

2 teaspoons castor oil

1 teaspoon black pepper oil

Directions:

Mix all ingredients well, then transfer into a spray bottle or spritzer. When you are ready to use, shake the bottle thoroughly each time, and generously spray the area that is currently infected, or the area you want to protect from infestation.

If you wish to use it as a repellent on yourself, simple spray your wrists and rub it around the back of your neck and behind your ears. This is not waterproof, so if you go swimming you will need to reapply.

Also reapply as needed.

Better Than Mesh
What you will need:

12 drops vanilla oil

8 drops cinnamon oil

½ cup water

1 tablespoon witch hazel

2 teaspoons castor oil

1 teaspoon black pepper oil

Directions:

Mix all ingredients well, then transfer into a spray bottle or spritzer. When you are ready to use, shake the bottle thoroughly each time, and generously spray the area that is currently infected, or the area you want to protect from infestation.

If you wish to use it as a repellent on yourself, simple spray your wrists and rub it around the back of your neck and behind your ears. This is not waterproof, so if you go swimming you will need to reapply.

Also reapply as needed.

Double Or Nothing

What you will need:

12 drops garlic oil

12 drops basil oil

½ cup water

1 tablespoon witch hazel

2 teaspoons castor oil

1 teaspoon black pepper oil

Directions:

Mix all ingredients well, then transfer into a spray bottle or spritzer. When you are ready to use, shake the bottle thoroughly each time, and generously spray the area that is currently infected, or the area you want to protect from infestation.

If you wish to use it as a repellent on yourself, simple spray your wrists and rub it around the back of your neck and behind your ears. This is not waterproof, so if you go swimming you will need to reapply.

Also reapply as needed.

Very Merry Holiday

What you will need:

12 drops citronella oil

8 drops lemongrass oil

½ cup water

1 tablespoon witch hazel

2 teaspoons castor oil

1 teaspoon black pepper oil

Directions:

Mix all ingredients well, then transfer into a spray bottle or spritzer. When you are ready to use, shake the bottle thoroughly each time, and generously spray the area that is currently infected, or the area you want to protect from infestation.

If you wish to use it as a repellent on yourself, simple spray your wrists and rub it around the back of your neck and behind your ears. This is not waterproof, so if you go swimming you will need to reapply.

Also reapply as needed.

The Real Deal
What you will need:

12 drops lemon oil

7 drops lemongrass oil

½ cup water

1 tablespoon witch hazel

2 teaspoons castor oil

1 teaspoon black pepper oil

Directions:

Mix all ingredients well, then transfer into a spray bottle or spritzer. When you are ready to use, shake the bottle thoroughly each time, and generously spray the area that is currently infected, or the area you want to protect from infestation.

If you wish to use it as a repellent on yourself, simple spray your wrists and rub it around the back of your neck and behind your ears. This is not waterproof, so if you go swimming you will need to reapply.

Also reapply as needed.

Spice Girl

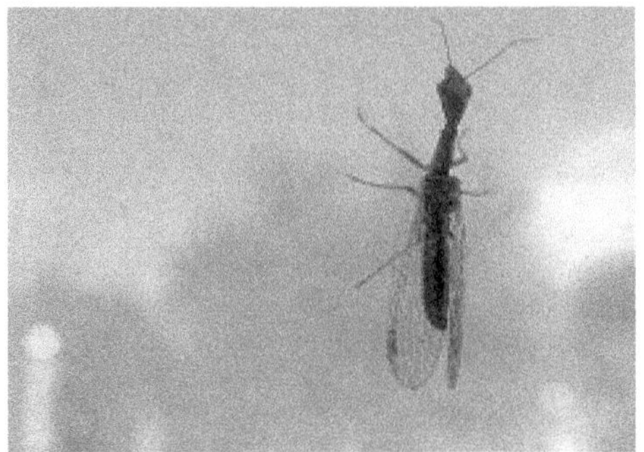

What you will need:

12 drops clove oil

1 teaspoon olive oil

½ cup water

1 tablespoon witch hazel

2 teaspoons castor oil

1 teaspoon black pepper oil

Directions:

Mix all ingredients well, then transfer into a spray bottle or spritzer. When you are ready to use, shake the bottle thoroughly each time, and generously spray the area that is currently infected, or the area you want to protect from infestation.

If you wish to use it as a repellent on yourself, simple spray your wrists and rub it around the back of your neck and behind your ears. This is not waterproof, so if you go swimming you will need to reapply.

Also reapply as needed.

Better-Fly Away

What you will need:

18 drops citronella oil

12 drops eucalyptus oil

½ cup water

1 tablespoon witch hazel

2 teaspoons castor oil

1 teaspoon black pepper oil

Directions:

Mix all ingredients well, then transfer into a spray bottle or spritzer. When you are ready to use, shake the bottle thoroughly each time, and generously spray the area that is currently infected, or the area you want to protect from infestation.

If you wish to use it as a repellent on yourself, simple spray your wrists and rub it around the back of your neck and behind your ears. This is not waterproof, so if you go swimming you will need to reapply.

Also reapply as needed.

That's the Ticket

What you will need:

1 tablespoon castor oil

1 teaspoon rubbing alcohol

½ cup water

1 tablespoon witch hazel

2 teaspoons castor oil

1 teaspoon black pepper oil

Directions:

Mix all ingredients well, then transfer into a spray bottle or spritzer. When you are ready to use, shake the bottle thoroughly each time, and generously spray the area that is currently infected, or the area you want to protect from infestation.

If you wish to use it as a repellent on yourself, simple spray your wrists and rub it around the back of your neck and behind your ears. This is not waterproof, so if you go swimming you will need to reapply.

Also reapply as needed.

Beetle Juice

What you will need:

12 drops citronella oil

1 teaspoon castor oil

½ cup water

1 tablespoon witch hazel

2 teaspoons castor oil

1 teaspoon black pepper oil

Directions:

Mix all ingredients well, then transfer into a spray bottle or spritzer. When you are ready to use, shake the bottle thoroughly each time, and generously spray the area that is currently infected, or the area you want to protect from infestation.

If you wish to use it as a repellent on yourself, simple spray your wrists and rub it around the back of your neck and behind your ears. This is not waterproof, so if you go swimming you will need to reapply.

Also reapply as needed.

Spider Swiffer
What you will need:

12 drops lemongrass oil

19 drops grapefruit oil

½ cup water

1 tablespoon witch hazel

2 teaspoons castor oil

1 teaspoon black pepper oil

Directions:

Mix all ingredients well, then transfer into a spray bottle or spritzer. When you are ready to use, shake the bottle thoroughly each time, and generously spray the area that is currently infected, or the area you want to protect from infestation.

If you wish to use it as a repellent on yourself, simple spray your wrists and rub it around the back of your neck and behind your ears. This is not waterproof, so if you go swimming you will need to reapply.

Also reapply as needed.

Crack Master

What you will need:

12 drops vanilla oil

7 drops lemon oil

½ cup water

1 tablespoon witch hazel

2 teaspoons castor oil

1 teaspoon black pepper oil

Directions:

Mix all ingredients well, then transfer into a spray bottle or spritzer. When you are ready to use, shake the bottle thoroughly each time, and generously spray the area that is currently infected, or the area you want to protect from infestation.

If you wish to use it as a repellent on yourself, simple spray your wrists and rub it around the back of your neck and behind your ears. This is not waterproof, so if you go swimming you will need to reapply.

Also reapply as needed.

It's a Pet Thing

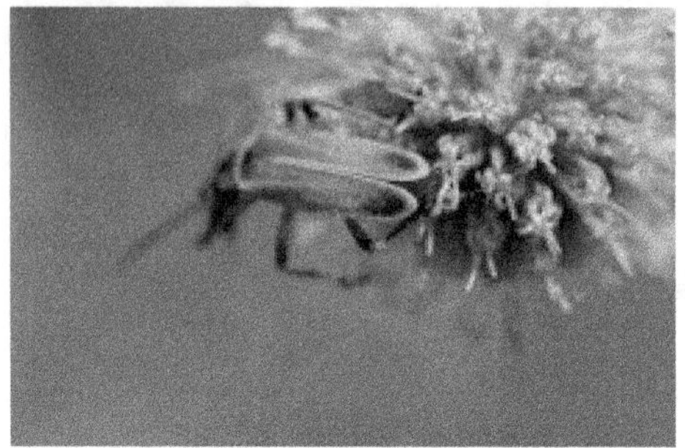

What you will need:

12 drops tea tree oil

9 drops clove oil

½ cup water

1 tablespoon witch hazel

2 teaspoons castor oil

1 teaspoon black pepper oil

Directions:

Mix all ingredients well, then transfer into a spray bottle or spritzer. When you are ready to use, shake the bottle thoroughly each time, and generously spray the area that is currently infected, or the area you want to protect from infestation.

If you wish to use it as a repellent on yourself, simple spray your wrists and rub it around the back of your neck and behind your ears. This is not waterproof, so if you go swimming you will need to reapply.

Also reapply as needed.

Kind of a Big Deal

What you will need:

12 drops peppermint oil

8 drops spearmint oil

½ cup water

1 tablespoon witch hazel

2 teaspoons castor oil

1 teaspoon black pepper oil

Directions:

Mix all ingredients well, then transfer into a spray bottle or spritzer. When you are ready to use, shake the bottle thoroughly each time, and generously spray the area that is currently infected, or the area you want to protect from infestation.

If you wish to use it as a repellent on yourself, simple spray your wrists and rub it around the back of your neck and behind your ears. This is not waterproof, so if you go swimming you will need to reapply.

Also reapply as needed.

Mist Miracle

What you will need:

12 drops lavender oil

8 drops eucalyptus oil

8 drops vanilla oil

½ cup water

1 tablespoon witch hazel

2 teaspoons castor oil

1 teaspoon black pepper oil

Directions:

Mix all ingredients well, then transfer into a spray bottle or spritzer. When you are ready to use, shake the bottle thoroughly each time, and generously spray the area that is currently infected, or the area you want to protect from infestation.

If you wish to use it as a repellent on yourself, simple spray your wrists and rub it around the back of your neck and behind your ears. This is not waterproof, so if you go swimming you will need to reapply.

Also reapply as needed.

The Fortress
What you will need:

12 drops vanilla oil

1 teaspoon sweet jojoba oil

½ cup water

1 tablespoon witch hazel

2 teaspoons castor oil

1 teaspoon black pepper oil

Directions:

Mix all ingredients well, then transfer into a spray bottle or spritzer. When you are ready to use, shake the bottle thoroughly each time, and generously spray the area that is currently infected, or the area you want to protect from infestation.

If you wish to use it as a repellent on yourself, simple spray your wrists and rub it around the back of your neck and behind your ears. This is not waterproof, so if you go swimming you will need to reapply.

Also reapply as needed.

Bug Barricade

What you will need:

18 drops citronella oil

12 drops cinnamon oil

½ cup water

1 tablespoon witch hazel

2 teaspoons castor oil

1 teaspoon black pepper oil

Directions:

Mix all ingredients well, then transfer into a spray bottle or spritzer. When you are ready to use, shake the bottle thoroughly each time, and generously spray the area that is currently infected, or the area you want to protect from infestation.

If you wish to use it as a repellent on yourself, simple spray your wrists and rub it around the back of your neck and behind your ears. This is not waterproof, so if you go swimming you will need to reapply.

Also reapply as needed.

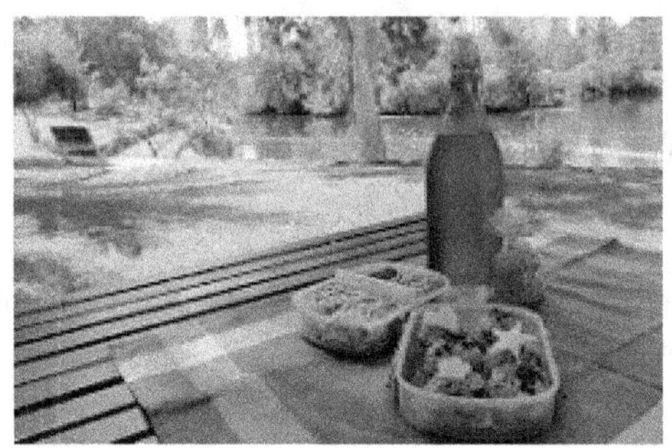

Shoo!

What you will need:

12 drops lemon oil

9 drops rosewood oil

½ cup water

1 tablespoon witch hazel

2 teaspoons castor oil

1 teaspoon black pepper oil

Directions:

Mix all ingredients well, then transfer into a spray bottle or spritzer. When you are ready to use, shake the bottle thoroughly each time, and generously spray the area that is currently infected, or the area you want to protect from infestation.

If you wish to use it as a repellent on yourself, simple spray your wrists and rub it around the back of your neck and behind your ears. This is not waterproof, so if you go swimming you will need to reapply.

Also reapply as needed.

Just Juice
What you will need:

14 drops ylang ylang oil

12 drops vetiver oil

½ cup water

1 tablespoon witch hazel

2 teaspoons castor oil

1 teaspoon black pepper oil

Directions:

Mix all ingredients well, then transfer into a spray bottle or spritzer. When you are ready to use, shake the bottle thoroughly each time, and generously spray the area that is currently infected, or the area you want to protect from infestation.

If you wish to use it as a repellent on yourself, simple spray your wrists and rub it around the back of your neck and behind your ears. This is not waterproof, so if you go swimming you will need to reapply.

Also reapply as needed.

When There is No Screen
What you will need:

12 drops citronella oil

8 drops cardamom oil

½ cup water

1 tablespoon witch hazel

2 teaspoons castor oil

1 teaspoon black pepper oil

Directions:

Mix all ingredients well, then transfer into a spray bottle or spritzer. When you are ready to use, shake the bottle thoroughly each time, and generously spray the area that is currently infected, or the area you want to protect from infestation.

If you wish to use it as a repellent on yourself, simple spray your wrists and rub it around the back of your neck and behind your ears. This is not waterproof, so if you go swimming you will need to reapply.

Also reapply as needed.

Better than Mesh
What you will need:

13 drops rose oil

1 teaspoon sunflower oil

½ cup water

1 tablespoon witch hazel

2 teaspoons castor oil

1 teaspoon black pepper oil

Directions:

Mix all ingredients well, then transfer into a spray bottle or spritzer. When you are ready to use, shake the bottle thoroughly each time, and generously spray the area that is currently infected, or the area you want to protect from infestation.

If you wish to use it as a repellent on yourself, simple spray your wrists and rub it around the back of your neck and behind your ears. This is not waterproof, so if you go swimming you will need to reapply.

Also reapply as needed.

Top Notch

What you will need:

13 drops vetiver oil

17 drops chamomile oil

½ cup water

1 tablespoon witch hazel

2 teaspoons castor oil

1 teaspoon black pepper oil

Directions:

Mix all ingredients well, then transfer into a spray bottle or spritzer. When you are ready to use, shake the bottle thoroughly each time, and generously spray the area that is currently infected, or the area you want to protect from infestation.

If you wish to use it as a repellent on yourself, simple spray your wrists and rub it around the back of your neck and behind your ears. This is not waterproof, so if you go swimming you will need to reapply.

Also reapply as needed.

Summer Solstice
What you will need:

12 drops orange oil

13 drops lemon oil

½ cup water

1 tablespoon witch hazel

2 teaspoons castor oil

1 teaspoon black pepper oil

Directions:

Mix all ingredients well, then transfer into a spray bottle or spritzer. When you are ready to use, shake the bottle thoroughly each time, and generously spray the area that is currently infected, or the area you want to protect from infestation.

If you wish to use it as a repellent on yourself, simple spray your wrists and rub it around the back of your neck and behind your ears. This is not waterproof, so if you go swimming you will need to reapply.

Also reapply as needed.

Buzzer
What you will need:

12 drops sage oil

19 drops clary sage oil

½ cup water

1 tablespoon witch hazel

2 teaspoons castor oil

1 teaspoon black pepper oil

Directions:

Mix all ingredients well, then transfer into a spray bottle or spritzer. When you are ready to use, shake the bottle thoroughly each time, and generously spray the area that is currently infected, or the area you want to protect from infestation.

If you wish to use it as a repellent on yourself, simple spray your wrists and rub it around the back of your neck and behind your ears. This is not waterproof, so if you go swimming you will need to reapply.

Also reapply as needed.

Breezy Afternoon
What you will need:

9 drops geranium oil

12 drops ylang ylang

½ cup water

1 tablespoon witch hazel

2 teaspoons castor oil

1 teaspoon black pepper oil

Directions:

Mix all ingredients well, then transfer into a spray bottle or spritzer. When you are ready to use, shake the bottle thoroughly each time, and generously spray the area that is currently infected, or the area you want to protect from infestation.

If you wish to use it as a repellent on yourself, simple spray your wrists and rub it around the back of your neck and behind your ears. This is not waterproof, so if you go swimming you will need to reapply.

Also reapply as needed.

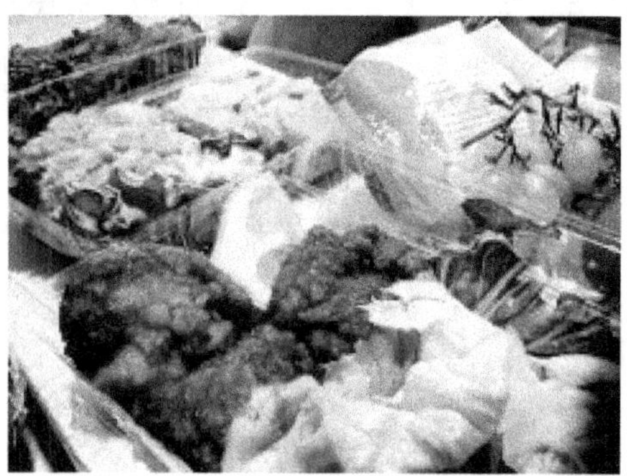

Wasp Stop

What you will need:

12 drops peppermint oil

12 drops citronella oil

½ cup water

1 tablespoon witch hazel

2 teaspoons castor oil

1 teaspoon black pepper oil

Directions:

Mix all ingredients well, then transfer into a spray bottle or spritzer. When you are ready to use, shake the bottle thoroughly each time, and generously spray the area that is currently infected, or the area you want to protect from infestation.

If you wish to use it as a repellent on yourself, simple spray your wrists and rub it around the back of your neck and behind your ears. This is not waterproof, so if you go swimming you will need to reapply.

Also reapply as needed.

Magic Guard

What you will need:

12 drops bergamot oil

13 drops sage oil

½ cup water

1 tablespoon witch hazel

2 teaspoons castor oil

1 teaspoon black pepper oil

Directions:

Mix all ingredients well, then transfer into a spray bottle or spritzer. When you are ready to use, shake the bottle thoroughly each time, and generously spray the area that is currently infected, or the area you want to protect from infestation.

If you wish to use it as a repellent on yourself, simple spray your wrists and rub it around the back of your neck and behind your ears. This is not waterproof, so if you go swimming you will need to reapply.

Also reapply as needed.

Chapter 2 – The Bigger Bombs

Mouse Be Gone

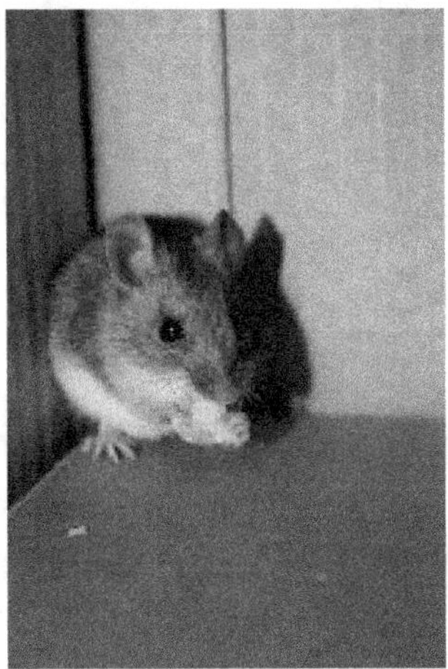

What you will need:

1 tablespoon peppermint oil

1 cup warm water

Cotton balls

Directions:

Combine all ingredients in a bottle and shake to mix well. When the solution is mixed, spray or pour generously on cotton balls. Place the cotton balls around your home, especially where you know the animals are getting in or like to hide.

You can also place these cotton balls along the wall to keep the internal visitors at bay. These balls will be effective for as long as the scent lasts – usually about 2 weeks.

Repeat as often as needed.

The Mousinator
What you will need:

1 tablespoon castor oil

1 tablespoon tobasco sauce

1 cup warm water

Cotton balls

Directions:

Combine all ingredients in a bottle and shake to mix well. When the solution is mixed, spray or pour generously on cotton balls. Place the cotton balls around your home, especially where you know the animals are getting in or like to hide.

You can also place these cotton balls along the wall to keep the internal visitors at bay. These balls will be effective for as long as the scent lasts – usually about 2 weeks.

Repeat as often as needed.

Leave it to the Cat
What you will need:

1 tablespoon laundry detergent

1 tablespoon vinegar

1 teaspoon peppermint oil

1 cup water

Cotton balls

Directions:

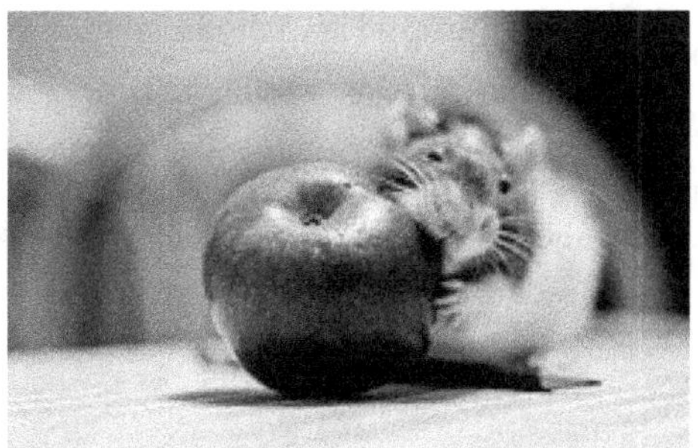

Combine all ingredients in a bottle and shake to mix well. When the solution is mixed, spray or pour generously on cotton balls. Place the cotton balls around your home, especially where you know the animals are getting in or like to hide.

You can also place these cotton balls along the wall to keep the internal visitors at bay. These balls will be effective for as long as the scent lasts – usually about 2 weeks.

Repeat as often as needed.

Rat Splat
What you will need:

1 tablespoon tobasco sauce

1 tablespoon white vinegar

2 teaspoons peppermint oil

1 tablespoon laundry detergent

Cotton balls

Directions:

Combine all ingredients in a bottle and shake to mix well. When the solution is mixed, spray or pour generously on cotton balls. Place the cotton balls around your home, especially where you know the animals are getting in or like to hide.

You can also place these cotton balls along the wall to keep the internal visitors at bay. These balls will be effective for as long as the scent lasts – usually about 2 weeks.

Repeat as often as needed.

No More Rats
What you will need:

1 tablespoon apple cider vinegar

1 tablespoon castor oil

1 tablespoon tea tree oil

1 teaspoon peppermint oil

Cotton balls

Directions:

Combine all ingredients in a bottle and shake to mix well. When the solution is mixed, spray or pour generously on cotton balls. Place the cotton balls around your home, especially where you know the animals are getting in or like to hide.

You can also place these cotton balls along the wall to keep the internal visitors at bay. These balls will be effective for as long as the scent lasts – usually about 2 weeks.

Repeat as often as needed.

Conclusion

There you have it, everything you need to know to protect your home from all kinds of pesky creatures that try to get in. You know you want to keep your home safe and secure from anything that you didn't invite to come inside, and what better way to do that than with your own non-toxic formulas?

Each and every one of these is highly effective against every kind of pest you can think of, so don't be shy – mix up as many as you want today. Mix and match to find the one you like the best, and your house is not only going to smell amazing, you are also going to be free of any pest.

Good luck!

FREE Bonus Reminder

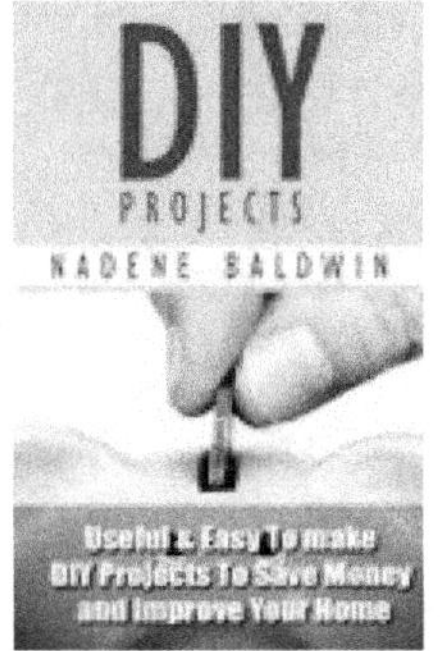

If you have not grabbed it yet, please go ahead and download your special bonus report *"DIY Projects. 13 Useful & Easy To Make DIY Projects To Save Money & Improve Your Home!"*

Simply Click the Button Below

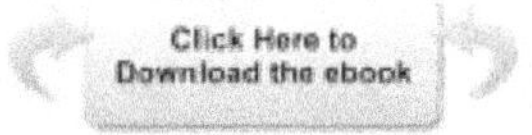

OR **Go to This Page**

http://diyhomecraft.com/free

BONUS #2: More Free & Discounted Books or Products

Do you want to receive more Free/Discounted Books or Products?

We have a mailing list where we send out our new Books or Products when they go free or with a discount on Amazon. Click on the link below to sign up for Free & Discount Book & Product Promotions.

=> Sign Up for Free & Discount Book & Product Promotions <=

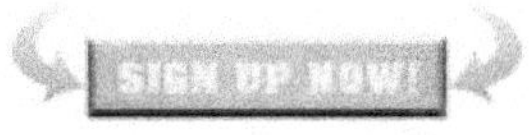

OR Go to this URL